FREQUENCIES THAT HEAL

AN EASY GUIDE TO CLEAR TRAUMA & LIVE JOYFULLY

DR. F. GRACE N.D.

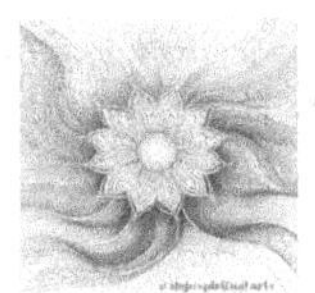

CONTENTS

INTRODUCTION

Life presents us with many challenges. We experience those challenges in so many different ways and are often in positions that prevent us from weathering the traumatic storms of life as gracefully as we wish we could. That's just life. But we **do not** need to exist in the negative vortex of dis-ease and pain. We can clear our trauma and live a life of joy. This is a fact.

I struggled with my traumas for many, many years. As a young woman, I wrestled with depression. I raised my daughters as a depressed mother, and my patterns became theirs. This knowledge created further guilt, knowing that they, too, would suffer. I chose a man who struggled with his emotional demons, and he passed negative patterns on to our girls. This is how long-term family trauma works. We tend to remain in familiar patterns, practicing what has become ingrained in our psyches. We are subjects of our own patterns.

I was young, but that never stopped me from contemplating and asking questions. I analyzed and observed the cycles I experienced and the choices I made. I asked myself questions, always seeking answers to help me understand how I arrived, believing that if I understood the journey through the trauma, I could somehow cure it. And while many insights came to me, there would forever be unknowns, or at least, answers that have not yet come.

My healing journey has been long. I have used, and still do use many natural modalities, including meditation, acupressure, Qigong, tapping (eft), Chinese herbs, rebirth, and many others. While these modalities have helped me live in happiness, it was the discovery of the power of frequencies that created profound shifts for me and my clients.

Shortly after becoming a Naturopathic Doctor, I started incorporating flower tinctures into my protocols. The subtle power was lovely. I began playing with recipes for different dis-eases my clients and I faced. I could provide relief gently, affordably, and even at a distance.

About this time, I began using a frequency machine and quickly found that I could recreate nearly any frequency I wanted. This promptly led to blending flower frequencies to create natural, effective, and easy-to-use frequencies and kits that my clients could carry in their phones and use as often as needed, wherever and whenever they needed them. It is a freeing discovery that has been a fantastic source of help for my clients.

I wrote this straightforward guide to provide a shorthand education on frequencies as a way to help others who want to live joyfully, spend as little time as possible reading and researching healing modalities and more time implementing them. Let's get started.

CHAPTER 1
FREQUENCIES

Frequency healing, also known as vibrational medicine. It's a holistic health practice that taps into the power of vibrations to balance one's health. Imagine your body is a finely tuned orchestra, vibrating at specific frequencies. When one instrument is out of tune, it throws off the whole symphony, leading to discordant notes, or various health issues. Frequency healing comes in like a skilled conductor, using sound, light, and electromagnetic fields to restore harmony and balance within your body's energy field.

In our modern world, stress-related and chronic illnesses are about as common as ice cream parlors; traditional medical treatments provide symptom relief, while ignoring the causes. But frequency healing offers a complementary approach by targeting the root cause—your body's energy fields. It's noninvasive and holistic, which is a fancy way of saying it's gentle and looks at the big picture.

With advances in technology and a better understanding of bioenergetics, we see that this isn't just some New Age nonsense. Research shows that specific frequencies can stimulate cellular repair, reduce inflammation, and clear up mental fog, proving that these thera-pies work. As we move towards personalized medicine, frequency healing stands out because it considers the unique vibrational signature of each individual. Whether you're in physiotherapy, mental health counseling, or palliative care, integrating frequency healing can enhance the effectiveness of your treatment plan, making it a versatile tool in our healthcare toolkit. So, let's keep those good vibrations coming!

ORIGINS

Picture ancient civilizations, where the Egyptians swayed in temples with sound and music to heal their ailments, and our Greek friend Pythagoras was all about those harmonious musical intervals. Over in China, they were mastering the art of Qigong and acupuncture, understanding the body's energy pathways long before it was common practice.

Fast-forward to the 20th century and scientists are stepping in with their remarkable tools. Enter Royal Rife with his Rife machine, targeting pathogens with specific frequencies like a superhero. And today? Technology and quantum physics are joining the party! Devices like PEMF therapy machines and sound therapy instruments are the latest stars, bringing therapeutic benefits that are simply dazzling.

So, here we are in the modern era, where frequency healing is not some ancient relic. It's making waves in contemporary medicine, showing us that sometimes the best way to heal is to feel those good vibrations.

THE SCIENCE OF VIBRATIONS AND FREQUENCIES

Everything, including your fabulous self, is made up of energy, vibrating like a cosmic dance party at specific frequencies. Quantum physics backs this up, telling us that matter is just a bunch of jiggling particles and energy fields. Every cell, tissue, and organ in your body has its own groovy beat, and when they're all in sync, you feel fabulous. But when stress, illness, or toxins crash the party, frequency healing steps in to get those natural vibrations back on track using sound waves, electromagnetic fields, and light to tune up your body's energy field and keep you humming along in perfect harmony.

. . .

Now, let's talk about the benefits. These therapeutic frequencies can make you feel like you're floating on a cloud of relaxation, zapping stress and boosting your mood and mental clarity faster than you can say "om." Sound therapy can take your brain from a frantic beta state to a chilled-out alpha or theta state, offering instant relief. Over time, bathing in these healing frequencies helps keep your body's energetic balance in check, warding off disease and keeping you youthful and vibrant. Even those stubborn conditions like chronic pain, fibromyalgia, and arthritis, which usually give conventional treatments a run for their money, show significant improvement with these therapies.

WHAT IS AN ENERGY FIELD?

Imagine yourself wrapped in a dynamic, shimmering electromagnetic bubble surrounding you and permeating every part of your being. That's right. This field is believed to extend beyond our physical bodies, mingling with the environment and encompassing multiple layers that vibe with different aspects of our physical, emotional, mental, and spiritual health. And let me tell you, this isn't just some ancient mysticism— modern science is catching on to what our ancestors have known for centuries.

The energy field comprises various subtle energy forms. When your energy field is balanced and flowing harmoniously, it supports your optimal health. However, disruptions or imbalances in this field can manifest as physical illness, emotional distress, or mental disturbances.

WHAT IS BIOENERGETICS?

Bioenergetics studies energy flow and transformation within living organisms, combining principles from biology, physics, and psychology. It explores how energy imbalances and blockages affect the body and how restoring proper energy flow promotes healing. On a cellular level, it involves processes like cellular respiration and ATP synthesis, while on a broader level, it examines the body's energy systems, such as chakras and meridians.

. . .

Techniques in bioenergetics aim to optimize these energy systems, enhancing the body's natural healing abilities. The human energy field, or aura, is a multi-layered field of subtle energy that surrounds and permeates the body and plays a critical role in overall health. This concept is essential in various spiritual and holistic healing traditions, which believe the aura reflects physical, emotional, mental, and spiritual states.

The aura serves several vital functions:
• **Protective Barrier**: Acts as a shield against negative energies and environmental influences that could harm the physical and subtle bodies.
• **Communication** facilitates the transmission of energy and information between individuals, their environment, and different layers of their being.
• **Health Indicator**: Reflects the state of physical, emotional, mental, and spiritual health. Practitioners of energy healing often assess the aura to detect imbalances or disruptions.
• **Healing and Balance**: When the aura is balanced and clear, it supports overall health and well-being. Energy healing practices aim to cleanse, repair, and strengthen the aura to promote healing.

While not visible to the naked eye for most people, the aura can be perceived through various means:
• **Clairvoyance**: Some individuals with heightened psychic abilities can see or sense the aura's colors and shapes.
• **Kirlian Photography** is a technique that allows us to view the energy field around objects, including parts of the human body, providing a visual representation of the aura.
• **Biofeedback Devices**: Some modern biofeedback and energy scanning devices claim to measure and visualize the aura, offering insights into a person's energetic state.

. . .

The human energy field, or aura, is a complex and dynamic field that plays a crucial role in maintaining health and well-being. It bridges a person's physical and spiritual aspects, reflecting their overall state of balance and harmony.

ROLE IN HEALTH

Energy Balance and Metabolism

Bioenergetics is fundamental to understanding metabolic disorders and conditions such as diabetes, obesity, and metabolic syndrome. Imbalances in energy production and utilization can lead to these chronic conditions. By targeting bioenergetic pathways, therapies can be developed to restore metabolic balance and improve one's health.

Cellular Health and Function

Healthy cells are the building blocks of a healthy body. Bioenergetics examines how energy production affects cellular health, including cell growth, repair, and apoptosis (programmed cell death). Efficient energy production supports cell function and longevity, while disruptions in energy flow can lead to cellular damage and diseases such as cancer and neurodegenerative disorders.

Physical and Mental Performance

Optimal energy production is crucial for both physical and cognitive performance. Individuals can enhance physical performance by optimizing their bioenergetic pathways. Similarly, brain health and cognitive function are deeply connected to efficient energy metabolism. Adequate energy supply to the brain supports mental clarity, focus, and resilience against stress.

BIOENERGETICS IN DISEASE PREVENTION AND MANAGEMENT

Chronic Disease Management

Many chronic diseases are linked to mitochondrial dysfunction and impaired energy metabolism. Addressing these underlying bioenergetic issues can help develop more effective treatments for conditions such as chronic fatigue syndrome, fibromyalgia, and cardiovascular diseases. Interventions that enhance mitochondrial function and energy production can improve the quality of life for people with these conditions.

Aging and Longevity

Bioenergetics plays a vital role in the aging process. As we age, mitochondrial efficiency typically declines, leading to decreased energy production and increased oxidative stress. Understanding and mitigating these changes through lifestyle interventions, nutritional support, and targeted therapies can promote healthy aging and extend lifespan.

Holistic and Integrative Health Approaches

Bioenergetics integrates well with holistic health practices that consider the body an interconnected system. Energy-based therapies, such as acupuncture, Reiki, and Qigong, align with bioenergetic principles by aiming to balance the body's energy flow. These practices, combined with insights from bioenergetics, can offer a comprehensive approach to health that addresses physical and energetic imbalances.

Research in bioenergetics continues to uncover new connections between energy metabolism and health, paving the way for innovative treatments and preventive measures. Advances in biotechnology and molecular biology are enhancing our understanding of manipulating bioenergetic pathways to optimize health. This knowledge leads to the development of novel therapies that can improve energy production at the cellular level, potentially transforming the treatment of many diseases and conditions.

PRINCIPLES OF FREQUENCY HEALING

Frequency healing is based on several fundamental principles that explain how vibrational energy interacts with the body's energy field.

Two basic concepts in frequency healing are resonance and entertainment.

Resonance

Resonance occurs when one vibrating system causes another to vibrate at the same frequency. Each organ and cell has a natural frequency, and harmony among these frequencies ensures optimal body function. Frequency healing employs external frequencies like sound waves, electromagnetic fields, or light to restore balance and promote healing by resonating with the body's natural frequencies.

Entrainment

Entrainment is the process by which two or more rhythmic cycles synchronize. In frequency healing, entrainment involves aligning the body's energy frequencies with an external rhythm or frequency. When exposed to a stable and harmonious frequency, the body's chaotic or disordered frequencies can begin to synchronize with the stable frequency, leading to a state of balance and coherence.

BENEFITS OF FREQUENCY HEALING

Physical Health

Pain Relief and Reduction of Inflammation

Frequency healing methods, such as PEMF (Pulsed Electromagnetic Field) therapy and sound therapy, have been shown to reduce pain and inflammation. These therapies improve circulation, enhance cellular repair, and decrease inflammatory markers, relieving arthritis, fibromyalgia, and injury-related pain.

Improved Cellular Function

By restoring the natural frequencies of cells and tissues, frequency healing can enhance cellular metabolism, increase ATP production, and support the body's natural repair processes. This leads to better overall health and faster recovery from illness and injury.

Stress Reduction and Relaxation

Exposure to harmonious frequencies can shift the brain from a beta state (associated with stress and active thinking) to alpha and theta states (associated with relaxation and meditation). This results in immediate stress relief, reduced anxiety, and improved mood.

Enhanced Cognitive Function

Techniques such as brainwave entrainment can improve mental clarity, focus, and cognitive performance. This benefits individuals with attention deficits, learning difficulties, or age-related cognitive decline.

Chakra and Energy Field Balancing

Many frequency healing practices focus on balancing the body's energy centers or chakras. Clearing blockages and harmonizing the energy flow can enhance spiritual well-being and promote inner peace and harmony.

Deepened Meditation and Spiritual Connection

Frequencies that resonate with higher states of consciousness can facilitate more profound meditation, spiritual insight, and a stronger connection to one's inner self. This experience enhances spiritual growth and a sense of connectedness with the universe.

Clearly, frequency healing can be profoundly helpful in many ways. Now let's focus on specific tools and how to use them.

CHAPTER 2
METHODS & MODALITIES

SOUND THERAPY

Sound therapy uses sound frequencies to bring the body's energy field into balance. By applying specific tones and vibrations, sound therapy can help to alleviate stress, reduce pain, improve sleep, and enhance overall health. This modality leverages the principles of resonance and entrainment to harmonize the body's energy and facilitate healing.

INSTRUMENTS USED IN SOUND THERAPY

Tuning Forks

Tuning forks are metal instruments that produce a pure, precise tone when struck. Each fork is tuned to a specific frequency, corresponding to different parts of the body or energy centers. Practitioners use tuning forks by placing them near or on the body to stimulate healing responses. The sound waves from the tuning forks help restore balance in the body's energy field and promote relaxation.

• A common practice is using a tuning fork tuned to 528 Hz, often called the "Love Frequency," which is believed to facilitate DNA repair and promote healing.

. . .

Singing Bowls

Singing bowls, often made of metal or crystal, produce resonant tones when struck or rubbed with a mallet. These bowls create rich, harmonic sounds that can deeply relax the mind and body. Crystal singing bowls, in particular, are tuned to specific notes corresponding to the seven chakras, helping to balance and align these energy centers.

• A practitioner may use a crystal singing bowl tuned to the note "C" to balance the root chakra, providing grounding and stability.

Gongs

Gongs are large, circular metal discs that produce a wide range of frequencies when struck. Their complex and powerful vibrations can induce a meditative state, reduce stress, and promote deep healing. Gong baths, where individuals are immersed in the sound waves of one or more gongs, are a popular form of sound therapy.

• During a gong bath, participants lie down while the practitioner plays the gong, creating an immersive sound experience that facilitates deep relaxation and healing.

Drums

Drums have been used for centuries in various cultures for healing and ceremonial purposes. The rhythmic beating of drums can alter brainwave states, promote relaxation, and release emotional blockages. Shamanic drumming, for example, uses repetitive rhythms to induce trance states and facilitate spiritual healing.

• A shamanic healer might use a hand drum to create a steady, rhythmic beat that helps a person enter a meditative state and promotes emotional and spiritual healing.

Chimes and Bells

Chimes and bells produce clear, high-pitched tones that can clear energy blockages and promote a sense of tranquility. These instruments are often used in meditation practices to signal a session's beginning or end and maintain focus.

• A practitioner might use a set of wind chimes to cleanse a room's energy or to signal transitions during a meditation session.

. . .

Vocal Toning

Vocal toning involves using the human voice to produce sustained vowel sounds or tones. This practice can directly influence the body's energy field, promoting healing and balance. By making specific sounds, individuals can target different areas of the body or energy centers.

• Chanting the vowel sound "Ah" can help open and balance the heart chakra, fostering feelings of love and compassion.

Mantras

Mantras are repetitive sounds, words, or phrases chanted or sung. From ancient spiritual traditions, mantras carry specific vibrational frequencies that can influence the mind and body. Repeating a mantra helps to focus the mind, induce relaxation, and align the energy field.

• "Om" is one of the most well-known and powerful mantras. Chanting "Om" is believed to connect individuals with universal consciousness and promote a sense of inner peace and harmony.

BENEFITS OF SOUND THERAPY

• **Stress Reduction**: The soothing sounds used in sound therapy can lower cortisol levels and promote relaxation, reducing stress and anxiety.

• **Pain Relief**: Sound therapy can alleviate physical pain by promoting relaxation and improving circulation, which helps to reduce inflammation.

• **Improved Sleep**: Sound therapy's calming effects can enhance sleep quality by helping individuals relax and enter deeper sleep states.

• **Emotional Healing**: Sound therapy can help release emotional blockages, promoting balance and well-being.

• **Enhanced Meditation**: Sound can deepen meditation practices, helping individuals achieve a state of inner peace and spiritual connection.

BIORESONANCE THERAPY

Electromagnetic Therapy

Electromagnetic Frequency Therapy (EMFT) is a treatment modality that uses electromagnetic fields to improve health and wellness. The basic principle of EMFT is to apply specific electromagnetic frequencies to the body to stimulate healing processes, alleviate pain, and promote overall well-being. This therapy is based on the idea that electromagnetic fields can influence cellular function, impacting physical and mental health.

PEMF devices generate electromagnetic fields that penetrate the body, affecting cells and tissues at a deep level. This therapy reduces pain and inflammation, enhances circulation, improves sleep quality, and accelerates the healing of injuries and fractures. Sports practitioners commonly use PEMF therapy to speed recovery.

Rife Machines are another form of EMFT, named after Dr. Royal Rife, who invented the technology in the early 20th century. Rife machines use specific frequencies of electromagnetic waves to destroy bacteria and viruses. The theory behind Rife machines is that each type of pathogen resonates at a particular frequency, and by applying the corresponding frequency, the pathogens can be disrupted and eliminated. While some practitioners have used Rife machines to treat chronic infections and cancer, the effectiveness of Rife's machine remains a topic of debate.

BENEFITS OF BIORESONANCE THERAPY

Allergy Treatment

Detecting and neutralizing the frequencies associated with allergens can help reduce allergic reactions and improve immune function.

Chronic Pain Management

This therapy is effective in managing chronic pain conditions such as arthritis, fibromyalgia, and back pain. By restoring the expected frequencies of affected tissues, bioresonance can reduce inflammation and alleviate pain.

Detoxification

Bioresonance can assist in detoxifying the body by identifying and neutralizing the frequencies of toxins and heavy metals.

Infection Control

Bioresonance can detect and treat infections by identifying the frequencies associated with pathogens such as bacteria, viruses, and fungi. Targeted frequencies can weaken or eliminate these pathogens, supporting the immune system.

Mental Health

Bioresonance therapy is also applied to mental health issues, including anxiety, depression, and stress. Balancing the electromagnetic frequencies of the brain can help improve mood and mental clarity.

LIMITATIONS AND CONSIDERATIONS

Scientific Controversy

Despite positive reports, bioresonance therapy remains controversial within the scientific community. Some critics argue that insufficient robust clinical evidence fully supports its efficacy, and more rigorous, large-scale studies are needed.

Individual Variability

The effectiveness of bioresonance therapy can vary significantly between individuals. The specific conditions, the patient's overall health, and the practitioner's skill can influence outcomes.

LIGHT AND COLOR THERAPY

Light and Color Therapy, or Chromotherapy, is a holistic healing method that uses light and color to alter a person's physical and emotional health. The underlying principle is that different colors and light frequencies can influence mood, energy levels, and physiological functions. Each color is thought to resonate at a specific frequency and wavelength, which can balance the body's energy centers, or chakras, and promote healing.

• • •

Chromotherapy involves using colors to treat various ailments and enhance overall well-being. Practitioners of Chromotherapy believe that colors can stimulate or calm the body's systems, depending on the specific needs of the individual. For instance, blue is considered a calming color that helps reduce stress and anxiety, while red is believed to be invigorating and can boost energy levels and circulation. The color green is associated with balance and harmony, making it helpful in promoting emotional stability. Chromotherapy can be applied through various means, such as colored lights, colored fabrics, or visualizations, to achieve the desired therapeutic effects.

Photobiomodulation (PBM), or low-level light therapy (LLLT), is another aspect of light therapy involving specific wavelengths of light to stimulate cellular function and promote healing. PBM uses red and near-infrared light to penetrate the skin and tissues, enhancing cellular energy production and reducing inflammation. This therapy is used for various medical conditions, including wound healing, pain management, and treating chronic conditions like arthritis and fibromyalgia. PBM has been shown to accelerate the healing of diabetic ulcers and reduce pain and stiffness in patients with musculoskeletal disorders.

Chromotherapy and Photobiomodulation represent noninvasive, complementary healthcare approaches that leverage light and color's therapeutic potential. While Chromotherapy focuses on the psychological and energetic effects of colors, PBM targets the physiological responses to specific light wavelengths.

FLOWER FREQUENCIES

Flower essences are alternative medicine that uses flower-infused water to address emotional and psychological issues. The concept of flower essences dates back to ancient cultures, but their modern development is primarily attributed to Dr. Edward Bach, a British physician, in the early 20th century.

Origins

The use of flowers for healing can be traced back to ancient civilizations. Indigenous cultures worldwide, including Native American, Australian Aboriginal, and ancient Egyptian societies, used flowers and plants for their medicinal and spiritual properties. These practices often involved creating infusions or flower extracts to address physical and emotional ailments.

Dr. Edward Bach developed the modern system of flower essences in the 1930s. Initially trained as a conventional physician and bacteriologist, Dr. Bach became dissatisfied with the focus on treating physical symptoms rather than the underlying emotional and psychological causes of illness. He believed that emotional imbalances were the root cause of many physical diseases.

Dr. Bach identified 38 flowers, each associated with specific emotional and mental states. He developed a method to prepare the essences by placing freshly picked flowers in pure water and allowing them to infuse under sunlight or through boiling. The resulting "mother tincture" was then diluted and preserved with brandy to create the flower essence remedies.

A flower frequency refers to the vibrational energy or resonance emitted by a flower, which is harnessed and used in flower essence therapy. Flower essences capture flowers' subtle energy or "frequency" to address emotional and psychological imbalances. This concept is that each flower has a unique vibrational pattern that can positively influence the human energy field.

Each remedy corresponds to specific emotional states. For example, Mimulus is used for fear of known things, and Impatiens is for impatience and irritability. Rescue Remedy combines five Bach flower essences (Rock Rose, Impatiens, Clematis, Star of Bethlehem, and Cherry Plum) designed to provide immediate relief in stressful situations. The Flower Essence Society developed California Flower Essences, which includes flowers native to California. It addresses a wide range of emotional and spiritual issues.

BENEFITS OF FLOWER FREQUENCIES

• Flower frequencies can help release emotional blockages, reduce stress, and promote emotional resilience.

• Many people use flower essences to support their spiritual practices, enhance their intuition, and foster a deeper connection with themselves and nature.

Below are a few examples of flower frequency 'recipes' I've created and their healing properties.

To see additional combinations (there are many), please visit my website at https://e-dojo-spiritualarts.com/

Mental Victory: BREAK-THROUGH BLOCKS

Chamomile - Calms panic and heightened anxiety.

Chrysanthemum - Soothes the deep fear of death and loss.

Elm - Balances insecurity around perfectionism and desire to please others.

Filaree - Soothes trivial concerns around daily life.

Cerato - For excessive anxiety, fear of failure, and over-dependence on others opinions.

Mental Balance: ENTER SELF-ACCEPTANCE

Chamomile - Restores calm.

Poison Oak - Subdues irritability, hypersensitivity, and hostility.

Impatience - Quells sudden angry outbursts and promotes tolerance.

Snapdragon - To control inappropriate anger and verbal abuse.

Willow - Soothes deep anger, bitterness, and resentment.

Fuchsia - To release deep-seated anger.

Mental Command: SELF-ACTUALIZATION

Olive - Raises energy level.

Pine - Lowers the need for perfection and self-blame.

Mustard - Lightens' black moods' and mood swings.

Elm - For overwhelmed by fear of failure.

Gentian - For lack of faith, dealing with setbacks.

Mental Liberation: ESTEEM YOURSELF
Buttercup - Affirms the inner sense of your true worth.
Calla Lily - Restores calm sense of self, releases confusion.
Evening Primrose - Absolves feelings of being unloved and unwanted.
Lotus - Open's Spirit pathway to conscious revelation.
Sage - Expands (self-)awareness of 'Sacred Being.'
Trumpet Vine - Opens pathways of self-expression through the word.

Today, flower essences are used worldwide as complementary therapies to support emotional and psychological well-being. They are often combined with other holistic practices such as aromatherapy, herbal medicine, and counseling. Flower essences are considered safe and non-toxic, making them suitable for people of all ages, including children and pets.

CHAPTER 3
CREATE YOUR PRACTICE

I t's clear how profoundly impactful frequency healing can be. But with so many modalities, knowing how and where to begin your frequency healing practice could feel overwhelming and challenging.

First, let me assure you that even little changes over time have transformative value. Begin at your pace, slowly incorporating different modalities, observing changes. You'll soon find the options that work best for you and with your lifestyle.

While you may want to continue your frequency education and take more time to learn about the different modalities and their benefits, there are options that you can incorporate into your daily life as soon as today.

SOUND THERAPY

• Find recordings of healing frequencies such as binaural beats or solfeggio frequencies. You can listen to these during meditation while working or before bed to promote relaxation and balance.

    • Invest in a singing bowl or a set of tuning forks. Spend a few minutes each day playing these instruments, focusing on the vibrations and their effect on your body and mind.

• Attend a local sound bath session or find online sound bath recordings. These sessions use instruments like gongs and crystal bowls to create a meditative and healing experience.

LIGHT THERAPY

Light therapy can seamlessly integrate into your daily life with the following practices:

• Spend time outside in the natural sunlight each morning to regulate your circadian rhythm and boost your mood.

• Use a light therapy lamp, especially during the darker months, to simulate natural sunlight and enhance energy levels.

• Use colored light bulbs or LED lights in your home to create a healing environment. For example, use blue light in your bedroom to promote calmness and better sleep or green light in your living room for balance and harmony.

BIORESONANCE

PEMF therapy devices are available for home use and are easy to integrate into home use:

• Invest in a PEMF Device. Use it for 20-30 minutes each day, preferably when you can relax and be still, such as before bed or while reading.

• Consistency is vital with PEMF therapy. To ensure you receive maximum benefits, set a specific time to use your device each day.

Combining meditation with frequency healing can deepen your practice:

• Use guided meditations that incorporate healing frequencies or binaural beats. These can help you reach deeper states of relaxation and enhance your meditation experience.

• Perform chakra meditations using corresponding frequencies or colors to balance your energy centers. Visualize each chakra being cleansed and energized by the specific frequency or color.

Transform your living space into a sanctuary for healing:

• Play soft, healing music or nature sounds in the background throughout the day.

• Use soft, colored lighting to create a calming atmosphere. Avoid harsh, artificial lights that can cause stress and fatigue.

• Complement frequency healing with essential oils that promote relaxation and well-being, such as lavender or eucalyptus.

PRACTICE REGULAR SELF-CARE

Integrate frequency healing into a broader self-care routine:

• Keep a journal to track your experiences with frequency healing and note any changes in your well-being.

• Practice mindfulness throughout the day to stay present and aware of how different frequencies affect you.

• Combine frequency healing with gentle physical activities like yoga or tai chi to enhance your body's energy flow.

FLOWER ESSENCES OR FREQUENCIES

Either tinctures or frequencies (such as the ones I create) are easily portable:

• Research flower essences to determine where to start

• Visit your local natural health store or look online and invest in a few essences.

• Visit my site https://e-dojo-spiritualarts.com to find custom blends that are immediately available and download them to your phone.

SEEK PROFESSIONAL GUIDANCE

If you're new to frequency healing, consider consulting with a practitioner specializing in sound therapy, PEMF therapy, or light therapy. They can provide personalized guidance and help you develop a customized plan.

Combining frequency healing with other holistic health approaches such as yoga, Reiki, and Emotional Freedom Techniques (EFT/ tapping) can create a synergistic effect that enhances overall well-being. Here's an example of a daily and weekly routine that integrates these modalities:

MORNING ROUTINE EXAMPLE: ENERGIZING AND BALANCING

Light Therapy and Yoga

• **Light Therapy:** Start your day with 10-15 minutes using a light therapy lamp or natural sunlight to regulate your circadian rhythm.

• **Yoga Session:** Follow this with a 20-30 minute yoga practice focused on energizing poses like Sun Salutations, Warrior Poses, and Tree Pose. Incorporate deep breathing exercises (Pranayama) to enhance the flow of energy.

• **Flower Frequencies** as needed.

Sound Therapy during Yoga

• **Healing Frequencies:** Play a soundtrack of solfeggio frequencies or binaural beats that promote balance and energy, such as 528 Hz (for transformation and DNA repair) or 396 Hz (for releasing fear and grounding).

MIDDAY ROUTINE: STRESS REDUCTION AND FOCUS

Meditation and Sound Therapy

• **Guided Meditation:** Spend 10-15 minutes in a guided meditation using binaural beats in the alpha wave range (8-12 Hz) to enhance relaxation and focus.

• **Tuning Forks:** Use tuning forks at specific frequencies that resonate with your chakras. Strike the forks and place them near your body or over specific chakra points to balance your energy centers.

EFT (Tapping)

• **Emotional Freedom Techniques:** Take a few minutes to practice tapping on acupressure points to address stress or emotional blockages. Focus on issues that may have arisen during the day, using affirmations to clear negative energy and promote positive feelings.

EVENING ROUTINE EXAMPLE: RELAXATION AND HEALING

Reiki Session

• **Self-Reiki or Practitioner Session:** Spend 20-30 minutes on a self-Reiki session or visit a Reiki practitioner. Focus on areas where you feel tension or imbalance, allowing the universal energy to flow and promote healing.

PEMF Therapy

• **PEMF Mat or Device:** Use a PEMF mat or handheld device for 20 minutes before bed. Choose settings that promote relaxation and deep sleep, such as low-frequency waves. Not only does this enhance overall relaxation, it can reduce pain and improve circulation.

Sound and Chromotherapy

• **Sound Bath:** Create a sound bath experience using singing bowls, chimes, or recorded sound baths. Allow healing sounds to wash over you, promoting deep relaxation and healing.

• **Chromotherapy:** Use soft, colored lights in your bedroom. Opt for calming colors like blue or violet to create a peaceful environment that supports sleep and relaxation.

WEEKLY ROUTINE: DEEP HEALING AND REFLECTION

Extended Yoga and Meditation Session

• **Chakra-Focused Yoga:** Dedicate a longer yoga session (60-90 minutes) to chakra-focused poses and meditations once a week. Use poses and breathwork that correspond to each chakra and incorporate color visualization for each energy center.

• **Crystal Healing:** Place crystals associated with each chakra (e.g., amethyst for the crown chakra, rose quartz for the heart chakra) around your mat or on your body during savasana (final relaxation pose).

Professional Reiki and PEMF Therapy

• **Reiki Practitioner:** Schedule a session with a Reiki practitioner for a more profound healing experience. This can help release deep-seated energy blockages and enhance overall well-being.

• **PEMF Therapy Clinic:** If you don't have a home device, visit a PEMF therapy clinic for a professional session. Professional devices may offer a broader range of frequencies and more powerful treatments.

Journaling and Reflection

• **Healing Journal:** Keep a journal to document your experiences with each modality. Reflect on any changes in your physical, emotional, and spiritual well-being. Note any emerging insights or patterns that can help you fine-tune your holistic health routine.

. . .

Incorporating these holistic practices into your life allows you to actively participate in your health and well-being. It encourages self-awareness and mindfulness and helps you understand how your lifestyle, emotions, and thoughts impact your health. By exploring and integrating these practices, you can develop a personalized approach to health that aligns with your unique needs and goals. Your healing journey will lead to a more balanced, vibrant, and joyful life.

CONCLUSION

n a matter of hours, you've learned far more about frequencies and their ability to heal than most people will ever know. You've also armed yourself with helpful tools that can change your life. The next step is up to you.

I wish you luck in your healing journey. It is your right to live joyfully, but you must take action. Stay in touch, and let me know how you progress. Reach out if you have questions or want to know more. I appreciate your time.

One last thing; If you think others should have access to wonderful healing frequencies, or you'd like to support the healing process of strangers, friends or family, please leave a 5-star review on Amazon. Share the opportunity to live joyfully with others. It's just good karma.

Also, visit my YouTube channel (https://www.youtube.com/@ floygrace6559) for a great selection of free frequency videos. Excuse the unpolished presentations—I'm just a sweet, esoteric grandma figuring out how to edit! But I've got your flower frequencies covered.

RESOURCES

Armstrong, A., & Armstrong, A. (2024, March 4). *Evidence-Based bioresonance*. Bicom Bioresonance Therapy | Bioresonance Therapy Information. https://bioresonancether apy.com/scientific-studies/are-there-evidence-based-studies-on-the-efficacy-of-bioreso nance-therapy/

Bioenergetics | Principal Investigator: Shilpa Iyer, Ph.D. (n.d.). https://bioenergetics.uark.edu/

DonovanHealth. (n.d.). *Healing the Body with Frequencies: The Basics Explained*. https://www. donovanhealth.com/blog/healing-the-body-with-frequencies-the-basics-explained

Franklin, D., & Franklin, D. (2023, September 25). A comprehensive overview of bioreso nance therapy. *Bioresonance and biofeedback discussion forum - Research scientific studies and forum for bioresonance therapy*. https://bioresonance.org/a-comprehensive-overview-of-bioresonance-therapy/

HHMGlobal, C. T. (2023, December 1). *The Science of Vibrations: Understanding how frequency healing works*. HHM Global | B2B Online Platform & Magazine. https://www. hhmglobal.com/health-wellness/the-science-of-vibrations-understanding-how-frequency-healing-works

Jrettig. (2024, March 27). Demystifying A Comprehensive Quantum Healing Explanation. *Quantum Healing Pathways*. Retrieved May 30, 2024, from https://quantumhealingpath ways.com/secrets-of-energy-healing/quantum-healing-techniques/quantum-healing-explanation/

King, R. (2024, May 7). *Frequency medicine: What you need to know*. Frequencell Inc. https:// vitalfield.com/frequency-medicine-what-you-need-to-know/

Martin, A. (2023, October 7). Exploring Frequency-Based Therapies: PEMF, RIFE, and the Science of Vibrational Healing - BlueSmartMiA. *BlueSmartMia*. https://bluesmartmia. com/exploring-frequency-based-therapies/

PEMF vs RIFE: How the Two Forms of Treatment Compare. (n.d.). HealthyLine. https://healthy line.com/blogs/blog/pemf-vs-rife-how-the-two-forms-of-treatment-compare

Rife machines and cancer. (n.d.). https://www.cancerresearchuk.org/about-cancer/treatment/complementary-alternative-therapies/individual-therapies/rife-machine-and-cancer

Russell, S. (2024, February 15). *Frequency healing*. Natural Healing Center - Grapevine, TX - Dr. Rodney Russell. https://drrodneyrussell.com/frequency-healing/

What are the 7 healing frequencies? Understanding sound therapy and its benefits - Yome Yoga. (n.d.). YOME YOGA. https://yogameditationhome.com/blog/healing-frequencies-sound-therapy-benefits

Wikipedia contributors. (2024, January 28). *Pulsed electromagnetic field therapy*. Wikipedia. https://en.wikipedia.org/wiki/Pulsed_electromagnetic_field_therapy